Causes & Treatment

of

Tonsils Infection

By

William kain

Table of Contents

Introduction

Causes and Treatment" is a thorough reference to comprehending the causes, signs, and available treatments for tonsil infections. Tonsil infections can be annoying, painful, and incapacitating, but they can be efficiently treated if you have the right understanding. The causes of tonsil infections will be covered in this book, including *bacterial, viral, environmental, and hereditary predispositions*. Also, we'll discuss the various forms of tonsil infections, such as acute, chronic, and abscessed tonsils. We will also explore the various tonsil infection therapies, ranging from at-home treatments and diagnoses to professional interventions like antibiotics and surgery. They are a crucial component of the immune system of the body and are composed of soft tissue resembling lymph nodes. The tonsils produce their white blood cells that fight infection, and because they are positioned in the back of the throat, they are well-suited to ward off and avoid infections. Tonsils can be classified as *palatine, adenoids, or lingual*. When you open your mouth, the palatine tonsils are the most noticeable; in contrast, the adenoids are located deeper and higher up in the throat, behind the nose. The lingual tonsil, the third kind, is likewise found at the base of the tongue. Living can occasionally be uncomfortable due to inflammation or swelling of the tonsils. Your tonsils may be swollen for some different causes, and the appropriate course of action will depend on the underlying issue.

Chapter 1

Tonsil Infections

*Definition of tonsil infections.

Tonsils are two masses of tissue that are found on either side of the back of the throat. Tonsil infections, often known as tonsillitis, refer to inflammation of the tonsils. The inflammation may be brought on by a bacterial or viral infection and is frequently characterized by symptoms including a sore throat, swallowing issues, fever, swollen tonsils, and occasionally white or yellow patches on the tonsils. Tonsil infections can be acute or persistent and can affect persons of any age, however, children are more frequently affected. Antibiotics, painkillers, and, in extreme circumstances, tonsil removal surgery are all possible forms of treatment.

*Typical signs of tonsil infections

Many symptoms can accompany tonsil infections, generally referred to as tonsillitis. The most typical signs are as follows:

*unwell throat

*red and swollen tonsils

*ache or trouble swallowing

*Tonsils may have white or yellow patches or a covering.

*Fever

*Headache

*An earache

*poor breath

*Fatigue\sChills

It's crucial to remember that not everyone will experience all of these symptoms and that each person may experience symptoms differently in terms of severity. It's crucial to consult a doctor for a diagnosis and treatment if you think you might have a tonsil infection.

*Types of tonsil infections

Tonsil infections come in a variety of forms,

The most prevalent type of tonsil infection is acute **tonsillitis,** which is characterized by tonsil inflammation brought on by a bacterial or viral infection. According to Medical News Today, **tonsillitis** happens when your tonsils are infected. A viral illness brought on by a **rhinovirus, adenovirus, influenza, or respiratory syncytial virus** is the most frequent cause. **Herpes simplex and Epstein-Barr** are two other viral infections that are less frequent. The most frequent cause of **tonsillitis** is a **viral illness**. Remember that a variety of things may play a role in the cause of your swollen tonsils. According to Healthline, the symptoms of tonsillitis can range from uncomfortable to chronic. Treatment is typically not necessary in acute situations. A doctor should be consulted, though, if you experience symptoms such as difficulty breathing, fever, muscle stiffness, or a sore throat that lasts more than two days. Antibiotics may occasionally be used as part of a severe case's therapy.

(Chronic tonsillitis)

This kind of tonsil infection happens when the tonsils get infected frequently over a long time. Tonsil stones are tiny, hard masses of germs and debris that can result in poor breath. They can be formed as a result.

(Peritonsillar abscess)

This is a complication of acute tonsillitis in which a pus-filled abscess develops around the tonsil. When pus gathers close to one of the tonsils, it develops into a *peritonsillar abscess (PTA)* Usually brought on by a bacterial infection, it can be very painful. A peritonsillar abscess can cause the following symptoms: acute *throat pain, difficulty opening the mouth or swallowing, Fever, discomfort in the ear, swelling of the neck's lymph nodes, and foul breath*. See a physician as soon as possible if you think you may have a peritonsillar abscess. To confirm the diagnosis, the doctor might do a physical exam and possibly prescribe imaging tests like a CT scan or ultrasound. Antibiotics are frequently prescribed to treat the infection, and the abscess may also need to be manually or surgically drained to allow the pus to drain out. To ease the discomfort, painkillers may also be provided. If the tonsils are chronically infected and causing recurrent abscesses, surgery may occasionally be required to remove them.

(Adenotonsillitis)

This is inflammation of the tonsils and adenoids, which are tiny masses of tissue at the back of the throat.

(Herpangina)

is a viral illness that results in tiny sores or blisters on the tonsils and the back of the throat.

* *infectious mononucleosis (mono),* is a viral infection that is spread by saliva droplets. After kissing or drinking from the same glass as someone who has the virus, you may become affected.

Tonsils that have an infectious mononucleosis may soften and swell. *Fever, headaches, and weariness* are among the additional common symptoms that the majority of virus-infected persons may encounter. These signs might not appear for four to six weeks following virus exposure, though. In reality, symptoms might occasionally resemble those of other medical diseases, Consequently, it is important to see a doctor if you are unsure of what is causing the infection. Typically, *a physical examination is used to make the diagnosis. They may check your tonsils for growth, see if your liver is bloated, or feel your lymph nodes in the front or rear of your* neck.

There is no particular treatment for infectious mononucleosis because it is brought on by a viral infection. Because of this, your doctor may urge you to rest, eat a healthy diet, and drink enough water.

(streptococcal pharyngitis) a bacterial infection that can result in severe tonsillitis and sore throat and, *if left untreated, develop into complications including rheumatic fever.* The bacteria streptococcus is a common cause of the ailment of **strep throat**. The illness typically manifests as a sore throat and is communicable. When a person with the streptococcus virus coughs or sneezes, the virus can spread by

droplets. Thus, touching doorknobs and other surfaces is a simple way to catch the illness, especially in the winter or early spring. When it comes to signs and symptoms, strep throat can cause red and swollen tonsils as well as several secondary symptoms like headaches, throat soreness, and difficulty swallowing. If breathing problems persist for longer than 48 hours, it's recommended to visit a doctor.

As a bacterial infection causes strep throat, treatment for it frequently involves *antibiotics like amoxicillin, cefadroxil, and cephalexin.*

*Tonsil stones

The openings in the tonsils are places where bacteria and other hazardous elements, **such as dead cells and mucus, can**. Your tonsils may become **calcified** or **hardened** when these **chemicals** become **lodged** there, giving them the appearance of *tiny stones*. Those with *chronic tonsil inflammation* are more likely to experience the development of these stones. Remember that the stones normally become noticeable as they grow in size, frequently showing up as white or yellowish spots on your tonsils, according to Healthline.

Although the specific mechanism by which tonsil stones develop is unknown, risk factors for their development include a lack of good dental hygiene or underlying illnesses like tonsillitis and persistent sinus problems. Moreover, the majority of tonsil stone cases show no symptoms. The anaerobic bacteria that are found in tonsil stones, which create smelly sulfides, may cause symptoms such as enlarged tonsils and bad breath. This is according to Medical News Today. You might also suffer a bothersome cough or a terrible taste in your mouth in addition to irritated tonsils and halitosis. Thankfully, at-home therapies are frequently a part of treatment. But if the stones are extremely big, your doctor might advise having the tonsils surgically removed (a procedure known as a **tonsillectomy**).

*Throat cancer

Your tonsils are not an exception to the rule that cancer cannot spread throughout the body.

When healthy tonsil cells undergo alterations that cause them to grow abnormally, Although the precise origin of tonsil cancer is unknown, recent scientific developments point to a relationship with the human papillomavirus (HPV). There are numerous examples of tonsil cancer where this STD has been found. But, if you use *alcohol or use tobacco*, you may also be at risk for tonsil cancer, tonsil cancer can develop even if your tonsils are removed since some tonsil tissues are left over after surgery. Remember that most tonsil malignancies are squamous *cell carcinomas*, with some being lymphomas. One approach to determine if you have tonsil cancer is to examine if one tonsil is bigger than the other. Another possible sensation is having something caught in your throat. Nonetheless, the illness may result in ear, throat, and mouth pain. Since they vary from person to person, symptoms might not be immediately apparent. But, if your tonsils are already huge, you may also experience poor breath and difficulties swallowing or speaking.

*underlying causes of tonsil infections.

Bacterial or viral infections are the most frequent causes of tonsillitis, often known as tonsillitis. Tonsil infections can, however, also be influenced by environmental variables.

(Air pollution) Breathing in polluted air can aggravate the throat and respiratory system, which makes it easier for bacteria or viruses to infect the tonsils.

(Allergies) Allergies can lead to throat irritation, making it simpler for germs or viruses to invade the tonsils.

(Cold weather) Cold weather can impair immune function and

make it simpler for germs or viruses to invade the tonsils.

(Indoor air quality) Tonsillitis can occur as a result of poor indoor air quality. This can entail being around dust, mold, or other allergens.

(Smoking) Smoking & smoke exposure can irritate the throat and respiratory system, which makes it simpler for germs or viruses to infect the tonsils. To reduce your risk of developing tonsillitis, practice good hygiene

habits and limit your exposure to certain environmental factors. You should see a doctor for a precise diagnosis and course of treatment if you suffer tonsil infection symptoms including fever, sore throat, or trouble swallowing.

*Tonsil infection is genetically predisposed to occur.

Genetic predispositions may contribute to tonsil infections, according to some data. A person's immune response may be impacted by specific genetic differences, making them more prone to infections or more likely to exhibit severe symptoms. For instance, a study that appeared in the journal Clinical Infectious Diseases discovered that specific genetic variants in the *IL-17* pathway were linked to a higher risk of recurrent tonsillitis. The immune system's response to infections is mediated by the *IL-17* pathway, and changes in this route may have an impact on a person's capacity to resist infection. a male or female individual's vulnerability to infections may be impacted by changes in the **TLR9** pathway, which is also implicated in the immunological response to infections. *Toxic tonsil infections can result from a variety of circumstances, but it's crucial to keep in mind that hereditary predispositions are just one of them.* Environmental factors and lifestyle choices are only two examples of additional elements that may be at play.

Chapter 2

Tonsil Infection Diagnosis

*Physical evaluations for tonsillitis

A medical expert will often examine the patient's throat, tonsils, and neck during a physical exam for a tonsil infection. To see the tonsils and throat more clearly during the examination, the doctor could employ a light and a tongue depressor. Moreover, they could palpate (feel) the neck to look for enlarged lymph nodes. The doctor will be on the lookout for symptoms of inflammation, such as tonsil swelling and redness, specifically for tonsil infections. Moreover, they could check the tonsils for pus or white patches. These symptoms might point to a bacterial infection like strep throat. The doctor may occasionally swab the patient's throat to obtain a sample of their secretions for laboratory analysis. This can aid in identifying the precise origin of the illness and directing the most suitable course of action. Overall, a physical examination is crucial for detecting and treating tonsil infections since it enables the doctor to determine the infection's severity and create a customized treatment strategy.

*Throat cultures to check for tonsillitis.

A diagnostic test called a throat culture can be used to find out whether a person's throat has bacterial or viral infections. Effective antibiotic treatment for tonsil infections depends on being able to identify the particular type of bacteria that is causing the infection. This information can be obtained from a throat culture.

A healthcare professional will use a cotton swab to collect mucus and bacteria from the back of the throat during a throat culture. After that, a laboratory is where the sample is grown in a unique culture medium. The bacteria will eventually multiply to the point where they can be seen under a microscope after some time. A throat culture can be used to monitor the efficacy of antibiotic therapy in addition to determining the type of bacteria that is causing the tonsil infection. After finishing an antibiotic course, a follow-up culture can be performed to confirm that the infection has been completely treated and to look for any bacterial strains that are resistant to antibiotics. It's important to remember that not all tonsil infections call for a throat culture, and a doctor will decide whether or not to order the test based on your specific case.

*Blood tests to diagnose tonsillitis

In most cases, blood tests are not required to identify a tonsil infection. Usually, the patient's symptoms and the results of a physical examination of the throat are used to make the diagnosis. *In some circumstances, medical professionals might request blood tests to support the diagnosis or track the progress of the infection.* Several blood tests may be requested in connection with a tonsil infection.

(Complete Blood Count (CBC) This examination counts the white blood cells present in the patient's blood. An infection may be indicated by an increase in white blood cell count.

(C-reactive protein (CRP) testing) This procedure gauges the amount of protein the liver secretes in response to inflammation.

Increased CRP levels could be a sign of an infection.

Using the *(mono spot test) a viral infection that can lead to tonsillitis is diagnosed as infectious mononucleosis.* It checks the blood for the **presence of Epstein-Barr virus antibodies.** *It's crucial to understand that blood tests cannot detect a tonsil infection on their own.* A healthcare professional should be consulted if you believe you may have a tonsil infection to receive a proper diagnosis and treatment plan.

Chapter 3

Tonsil Infection Treatment Alternatives

*Tonsil infection home remedies

A sore throat, difficulty swallowing, and other bothersome symptoms can result from tonsil infections, commonly known as tonsillitis, which can be brought on by bacterial or viral infections. Home remedies can aid in symptom relief and recovery even though they may not be able to treat the infection.

(Gargling) with warm water and a teaspoon of salt will help to reduce swelling and improve discomfort. Do this several times each day.

(Warm liquids to sip on) Warm drinks, such as soup or tea, might ease throat discomfort.

(Honey) Honey has antimicrobial characteristics and can help

relieve symptoms when added to warm tea or water.

(Rest) Obtaining enough sleep and drinking lots of water might aid the body in battling the infection and advancing healing.

Use a*(humidifier)* to moisten the throat and relieve irritation, or spend some time in a steamy bathroom.

(Garlic) Supplementing with garlic or ingesting raw garlic may help strengthen the immune

system and fend against infection. It's crucial to remember that you should consult a doctor if your symptoms get worse or last longer than a few days. Your healthcare practitioner may also suggest antibiotics or other medical treatment if you have frequent tonsil infections or other serious symptoms.

*Operating on the Tonsils

An operation called a **(tonsillectomy)** involves removing the tonsils from the back of the throat. The two tiny glands known as the tonsils, which are situated at the back of the throat and function to help fight infections, can occasionally become infected or grow, which can interfere with speech, swallowing, and breathing. *The patient will typically be given general anesthesia during a tonsillectomy, and the doctor will remove the tonsils with a knife or another instrument. Usually, the treatment lasts between 30 and 45 minutes, and the patient can leave on the same day.* The patient can suffer some throat irritation or pain following surgery and may need painkillers to treat it. A painful throat and difficulty swallowing for a few days after the treatment are other frequent side effects for patients.

It's crucial to adhere to the doctor's recommendations for post-operative care, which may include resting, drinking plenty of water, and staying away from particular foods and activities. Tonsillectomy is a routine surgery that is generally regarded as safe, but there are potential hazards, including bleeding and infection, as with any surgical procedure. It is crucial to talk with a doctor about the procedure's advantages and disadvantages before deciding whether it is the best course of action for the patient's particular circumstances.

*Tonsil removal using laser (tonsillectomy)

An operation to remove the tonsils with a laser is called a

laser tonsillectomy, often referred to as a laser-assisted tonsillectomy or laser tonsil ablation. *The classic tonsillectomy includes removing the tonsils by cutting or scraping them out with a knife or other surgical implements.* This method is frequently used as an alternative, A laser is used by the surgeon to cut away the tonsil tissue during a laser tonsillectomy. The tissue is heated by the laser until it vaporizes, at which point it can be suctioned away or removed using other tools. In addition to minimizing pain and discomfort after surgery, the use of the laser can assist reduce bleeding during the process. *If a person has sleep apnea, recurrent or chronic tonsillitis, or any other ailment that affects the tonsils*, a laser tonsillectomy may be advised. To find out if this surgery is the best option for you, speak with a trained healthcare practitioner. *It's crucial to keep in mind that not all people are excellent candidates.*

*Tonsillitis caused by rheumatism.

The heart, joints, and central nervous system can all be impacted by the dangerous inflammatory illness known as rheumatic fever. An aberrant immune response to an untreated or insufficiently treated group is what causes it. strep throat. *Tonsillitis, often known as rheumatic fever, is the infection of the tonsils.* Rheumatic fever-related tonsillitis *symptoms can include a painful throat, swallowing issues, fever, swollen tonsils, and uncomfortable lymph nodes in the neck.* There may also be additional signs of rheumatic fever, such as joint discomfort, fever, and a rash. You should consult a doctor as soon as you can if you think you or someone you know might have tonsillitis brought on by rheumatic fever.

Antibiotics to treat the underlying streptococcal infection as well as anti-inflammatory drugs to treat symptoms and stop additional problems are possible forms of treatment. Tonsillectomy, or the removal of the tonsils, may be required in several circumstances.

*antibiotic to treat tonsillitis

The type of bacteria causing tonsil infections (tonsillitis), the severity of the symptoms, and the patient's medical history all play a role in the selection of antibiotics.

*The most common kind of bacterial tonsillitis is treated with

(penicillin). The common cause of tonsillitis, streptococcus bacteria, is resistance to penicillin.

Another **penicillin** *that is occasionally recommended for tonsillitis is* **amoxicillin.**

*Erythromycin, clarithromycin, and azithromycin are among the antibiotics known as **(macrolides).** In patients who are allergic to penicillin, macrolides are utilized as a substitute.

*If a patient has a penicillin allergy, *(cephalosporin medicines)* may be administered for tonsillitis. Remember that only **bacterial tonsillitis** responds well **to antibiotic treatment; viral tonsillitis does not**. Before recommending an antibiotic, a doctor must determine whether a **virus** or **bacterium** is to blame for **tonsillitis.** Antibiotics should also be taken exactly as directed and for the whole duration of the treatment course, even if symptoms improve.

Chapter 4

Treating Tonsil Infections

*Hydrate and Sleep

Treatment of a tonsil infection involves rest and fluids. Sore throat, fever, exhaustion, and trouble swallowing are just a few of the symptoms that can be brought on by tonsil infections. Obtaining enough sleep can aid in the body's ability to fight off illness and hasten the healing process. Drinking enough water is also important since it can keep your throat moist and ease inflammation brought on by the illness. The removal of toxins from your body can also be aided by drinking lots of water and other liquids like tea or broth. You can treat a tonsil infection in various ways besides resting and drinking plenty of fluids. *To help with pain relief and fever reduction, these may include taking over-the-counter painkillers like acetaminophen or ibuprofen.* For throat comfort, you might also try gargling with warm salt water. It is crucial to get medical assistance from a healthcare expert if your tonsil infection is severe or does not get better with home care.

*How tonsil infections should be avoided

The following actions can be taken to avoid tonsil infections

(Maintain excellent hygiene)

Frequent hand washing and avoiding contact with those who have tonsillitis or sore throats can help stop the spread of infections.

(Drink lots of water)and keep yourself hydrated to keep your throat moist and lower the chance of infections.

Stay away from *(smoking and passive smoking).* Smoking can irritate the tonsils and increase the risk of tonsillitis. Tonsil infections can be prevented by not smoking or being around smoke.

(Adopt a healthy lifestyle) Consuming a well-balanced diet, getting adequate sleep, and lowering your stress levels can all help to strengthen your immune system and lower your risk of tonsil infections.

(Safe sexual behavior) is important because some tonsil infections, like strep throat, can be transmitted through sex.

Using condoms and other safe sexual practices can help lower the chance of contracting illnesses.

(Be immunized) Immunizations, such as the HPV vaccine or the flu shot, can help prevent some tonsil infections. *Talk to your doctor about additional preventive measures*, such as a tonsillectomy or prophylactic antibiotic use, if you suffer from tonsil infections frequently.

Chapter 5

Lifestyle Modifications to Reduce Tonsil Infections

*The impact of diet and nutrition on tonsillitis

Maintaining a healthy, balanced diet is crucial if you have a tonsil infection since it will strengthen your immune system and encourage healing.

(Get hydrated) To keep your body hydrated and ease a painful throat, consume plenty

of water, herbal teas, and warm broths.

(Concentrate on nutrient-dense foods) Fill up on fresh fruit and vegetables to provide your body with the vitamins and minerals it needs. **Citrus fruits, berries**, and **leafy greens** are examples of foods high in **vitamin C** that can help strengthen your immune system.

(Avoid irritants) Foods and drinks that are **spicy, acidic**, or

carbonated might aggravate your **sore throat** and **exacerbate** it. Stay away from these items and choose instead mild, easily digestible ones.

(Including probiotics) Foods **like yogurt** and **kefir** that contain helpful bacteria can help your body fight off infection and support your immune system.

(Get enough sleep) Sleep is essential for your body's ability to recuperate. Try for 7-8 hours

of sleep per night, and stay away from strenuous activities that can exacerbate your symptoms.

*Hygiene precautions for tonsillitis

Tonsil infections, like tonsillitis, are frequently brought on by viruses or bacteria and can spread quickly. It's critical to maintain adequate cleanliness to lower the possibility of a tonsil infection forming or spreading.

Wash your hands frequently. It's important to wash your hands frequently, especially before and after using the restroom, eating, or touching your face. This may aid in halting the spread of pathogens that can result in tonsillitis. ***While coughing or sneezing, use a tissue to cover your mouth and nose***. After using the tissue once, ***discard it***. This may aid in halting the spread of pathogens that can result in tonsillitis.

Never share utensils or personal goods with someone who has a tonsil infection. This includes glasses, cutlery, and other objects. This may aid in halting the spread of pathogens that can result in tonsillitis.

Using salt water to gargle Gargling with salt water helps ease a sore throat and lessen tonsil inflammation. Gargle for 30 seconds with a mixture of 8 ounces of warm water and 1/2 teaspoon salt before spitting it out.

Keep yourself hydrated Consuming lots of liquids can keep the throat moist and lower the chance of tonsillitis.

Avoid smoking and exposure to secondhand smoke because both can irritate the throat and raise the possibility of tonsillitis. Stay away from smoking and passive smoking.

Use mouthwash, floss your teeth every day, and brush your teeth twice a day to help limit the number of bacteria in your mouth that can lead to tonsil infections. If you have symptoms of a tonsil infection, such as a sore throat, fever, trouble swallowing, or swollen tonsils, you should see a doctor every once. They can suggest suitable medical care and additional sanitary precautions to take.

In conclusion

tonsil infections can be an ailment that affects people of all ages and cause them pain and discomfort. *Its signs and symptoms, which can include a sore throat, fever, swallowing issues, and swollen tonsils, can be brought on by viruses or bacteria.* Depending on the underlying cause and severity of the problem, there may be several treatment options for tonsil infections. *More severe infections would need prescription antibiotics or possibly surgical removal of the tonsils, while milder cases might get better on their own with rest and over-the-counter painkillers.* Good hygiene practices like routine hand washing, avoiding direct contact with ill people, and receiving vaccinations against certain viruses can all help prevent tonsil infections.

It's critical to see a doctor if you think you could have a tonsil

infection to ascertain the underlying reason and the best course of action. The majority of tonsil infections can be adequately controlled and treated with the right care and attention.